Take a Bite Out of Pain

A Journey to Overcoming
Temporomandibular Joint Disorders (TMD)

Mayoor Patel, DDS, MS & Sara Berg

This book is not intended as a substitute for the medical advice of any healthcare provider. The reader should regularly consult a healthcare provider in matters relating to his/her health, particularly to any symptoms that may require a diagnosis or medical attention. This book was written for educational purposes NOT for a diagnosis. For proper medical advice, please contact your healthcare provider.

© 2017 Mayoor Patel, DDS, MS and Sara Berg.
All rights reserved.
ISBN 978-1-365-61624-2

Table of Contents

Acknowledgement..6

Introduction...8

What is Pain?..10

The Many Masks of TMD.....................................12

- Neck and Shoulder Pain...........................15

- Headaches..16

- Pain or Pressure Behind the Eyes.............18

- The Sinuses..20

- Ear Pain...22

- Facial Pain...25

Pain in Children and Teens..................................27

The TMD Connection..32

- Connecting TMD and Tinnitus.................35

- Headaches and Migraines........................37

- Jaw Pain and Clicking............................39

- Misdiagnosing Fibromyalgia...................43

Causes of TMD..46

Treatment Options for TMD................................49

Watch What You Eat...61

The Connection Between Pain and Sleep...........................65

Case Studies……..…………………………………………...69

Alternative TMD Relief…..……………………………………85

Meet the Authors…………...…………………………………88

Dear Reader,

We wrote this book for you. Yes, you! Now, why would we think of you for a book? Because pain can include a variety of conditions, and we want to make sure you fully understand such a complex symptom. From headaches to temporomandibular disorders (TMD), pain is a shared symptom.

If you bought (or were given) this book, congratulations! You are now one step closer to understanding your pain. We've included everything you need to know—from signs, symptoms and causes, to conditions and treatment options. Use this book for a better comprehension of your symptoms and next steps in the journey to treatment. You'll even find a couple success stories!

Please take the time to read this book and pass it on to your friends and family. We hope this book helps you find a cure to your pain, and we look forward to hearing how you've used this book along the way.

All the Best,

Dr. Mayoor Patel

An Introduction to TMD

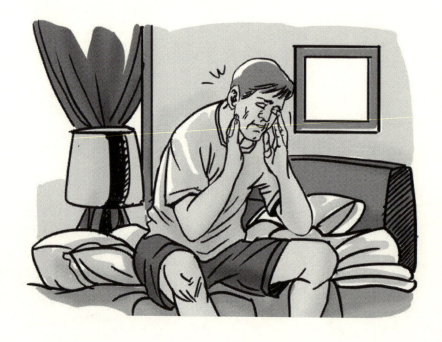

"One of the principle qualities of pain is that it demands an explanation." Canadian Poet, Anne Carson.

Have you ever experienced some sort of pain, whether it is in the front, side, or back of your head or neck, and simply brushed it off as nothing? Didn't think so. Pain does exactly what Canadian poet, Anne Carson says--it demands an explanation or some sort of reason why it is occurring.

If you are experiencing pain in your jaw or what seems like a regular headache, you won't just sit idly by as the pain is pounding in your head. No, you would get up, take medicine or visit your doctor.

Ignoring pain would simply be a waste of time, which is why finding the underlying cause to your nagging or constant pain is essential to helping you continue on with your day-to-day tasks.

Pain should not be accepted at face value. It is such a complex and complicated experience that is tuned by your brain--it triggers every painful sensation. So, are we just supposed to think pain away? No, absolutely not.

If you think of pain as a singular cause you won't get the answer you are looking for. Pain is almost never caused by a singular problem, which we will get into later on in this book.

What is Pain?

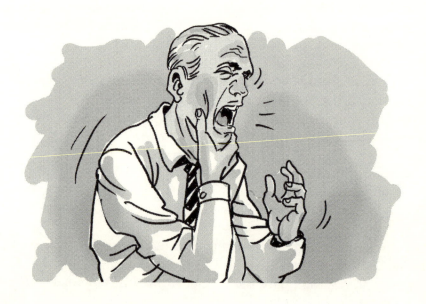

"Pain has a way of clipping our wings and keeping us from being able to fly...and if left unresolved for very long, you can almost forget that you were ever created to fly in the first place."

– WM. Paul Young, *The Shack*

This question almost seems like it needs an open-ended response. I think of it like Shakespeare when he states, "What's in a name? That which we call a rose by any other name would smell as sweet." No matter what you call pain; it is still uncomfortable and irritating.

In medicine, pain relates to a sensation that hurts. If you are experiencing pain, you feel discomfort, distress, and even agony depending on the severity of it. It can be steady and constant, causing an ache, or it can be a throbbing, pulsating pain. Your pain can even have a pinching or stabbing sensation. Any way you look at it, pain is uncomfortable and treatment is necessary.

When it comes to pain, there are two main types:

- **Acute Pain** - this can be intense and short-lived, and might be an indication of an injury. When the injury heals, the pain usually will go away.
- **Chronic Pain** - this sensation lasts much longer than acute pain and can be mild or intense (severe). Unlike acute pain, chronic pain does not go away without help.

Pain is not a reliable sign of what is going on--it might only be one factor in your condition that has lead you to seek further insight from a doctor or dentist. Chronic pain is like a witch's brew in the way that there are different factors that could be leading to the pain you are experiencing.

After all, according to Lorimer Mosely, "The biology of pain is never really straightforward, even when it appears to be." Now that we have a better understanding of pain, let's dive into pain and the many masks of temporomandibular joint disorder (TMD).

The Many Masks of TMD

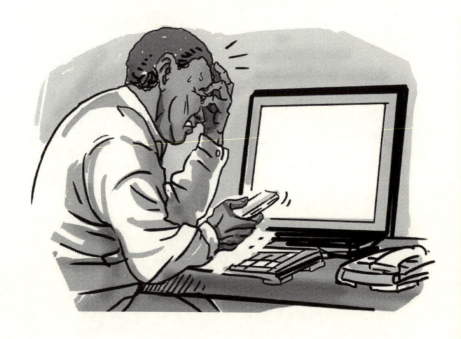

"The greatest evil is physical pain." - Saint Augustine

TMD is the abbreviated version of Temporomandibular Joint Disorder. However, we also often refer to this condition as temporomandibular joint dysfunction, or TMJD. It's a mouthful, but it has a very simple definition. TMD comes into play when difficulties arise with the jaw, jaw joint, ligaments, tendons and surrounding facial muscles.

These joints and muscles are very important for day-to-day life due to the fact that they play a crucial part in talking and chewing. Without the proper function of the jaw and jaw joint, everyday becomes a struggle. Pay close attention to the causes and symptoms of TMD so that, if need be, you are able to contact a doctor for assistance.

What makes TMD a tricky condition is the many masks it is often found wearing. Many people suffer from recurring head, face, neck, or jaw pain. However, it seems as if many can't seem to find help. They may even have been told it is all in their head and there is nothing that can be done to fix the pain.

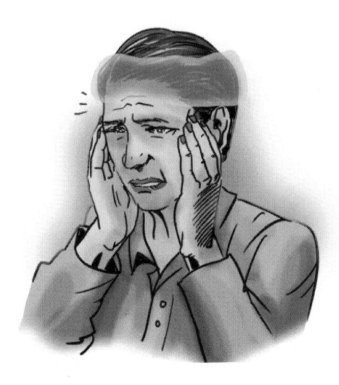

With many people being victims of unresolved chronic pain following car accidents or other forms of trauma, it is important to find a proper diagnosis to help eliminate or reduce chronic pain.

The temporomandibular joint (TMJ) is the most complicated joint in the body. When damage occurs to the TMJ, it can be noticed through early clicking or popping sounds during jaw movement, just to name a few signs.

Early detection can help to prevent more serious problems from developing because chronic pain can occur with TMD. For this reason, it is important to get treatment immediately.

We previously touched base on the idea that pain isn't just a singular cause. Instead it has a multitude of causes, which is the same for TMD--it is not just a single disorder. It is actually a group of painful conditions that can affect your jaw joint and chewing muscles.

Because the muscles in your face and jaw are intertwined, if your jaw is misaligned, it can lead to a series of problems from your head to your back and beyond. Let's take a look at a few different places chronic pain can occur and its relationship to TMD.

Neck and Shoulder Pain

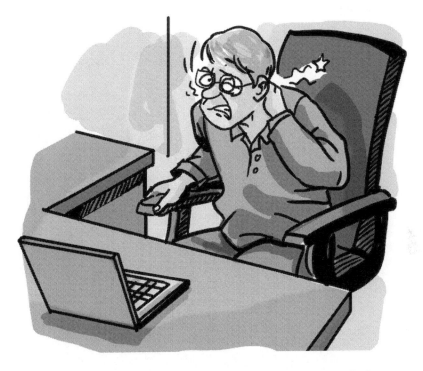

If your lower jaw does not close evenly it can create pain in your neck and shoulders. And when the jaw muscles don't properly function, the surrounding tissue may experience chronic stress, pain and swelling. Since your jaw runs in front of one ear to the other, as well as interacts with muscles in the neck, symptoms of jaw distress may surface in the neck and shoulders.

If you are experiencing unexplained pain in your neck and/or shoulders, you may be suffering from TMD. Because of the complex anatomic, neurological and physiological relationships within your head and neck, the symptoms of TMD can appear to be those of other diseases. For this reason, it is important to visit a dentist that is educated/trained in this area as soon as possible for a proper diagnosis.

Headaches

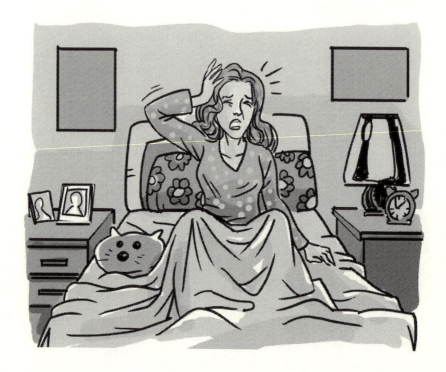

A misaligned jaw joint can cause the muscles in your face to constantly work hard leading to long periods of contraction, which, in turn, can create tension or pressure from the working muscle fibers.

When you are experiencing tension in your jaw, neck or shoulders, the muscles can squeeze the blood vessels and prevent the muscle metabolites from being excreted. This can cause more irritation to the muscles and nerve increasing your experience of pain.

Tension headaches and migraines are a common symptom of TMD, as well as teeth grinding. Migraine sufferers are often misdiagnosed because their doctor does not realize the issue can be resolved with TMD treatment. Many studies have shown that in chronic headache sufferers, a component of the TMJ is a contributor in patients not getting their condition resolved.

Pain or Pressure Behind the Eyes

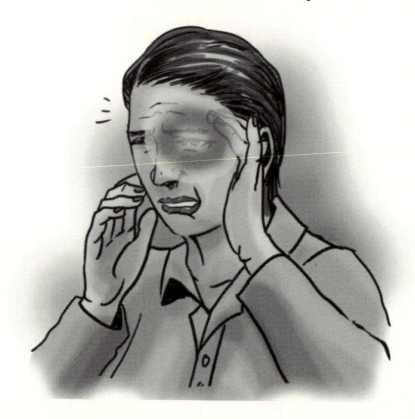

Do you feel a stabbing pain behind your eyes that makes it hard to concentrate? Or maybe you are experiencing pressure on your sinuses that makes you think you are allergic to everything? Even the slightest touch to your cheeks leaves you cringing. But why?

It is widely known that if you experience pain in your face, you likely have a problem elsewhere such as your eyes. However, most never reach the conclusion that your eye pain is related to TMD. For those who have a poorly aligned bite or missing teeth, health related problems such as facial or jaw pain could become more pronounced.

A bad bite in some patients may place strain in muscles that, in turn, will affect the placement of the jaw and the surrounding muscles. This imbalance in the bite-jaw-muscle relationship is what causes facial pain or pain behind the eyes. This can occur because the jaw muscles are working harder to bring the teeth together, which strains the surrounding jaw muscles.

If you are experiencing any of these symptoms, you may be suffering from TMJ disorder, a painful condition that is often mistaken for those recurring headaches and jaw pain.

The Sinuses

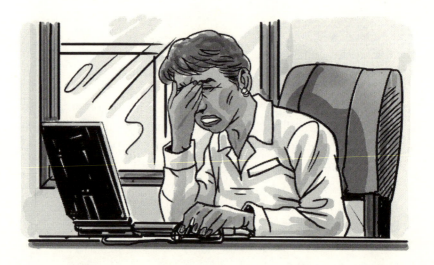

That's right! Your sinuses can be directly influenced by your TMD. When you suffer from TMD, you can also experience pain in your sinuses and other symptoms that can often be mistaken for a cold, chronic sinusitis and other infections.

However, it could be TMD because of the complaint of pain and pressure in the sinuses—even though there is no presence of a sinus disease, infection or inflammation. This is considered referred pain, which means the site of the symptoms is not the origin of it--what an interesting concept! As a result, you may begin to rethink past symptoms that you might not have been able to find the source of.

Your jaw muscles can refer pain to the sinus region, making a diagnosis difficult. Muscles that are tight, inflamed, and fatigued due to overuse behaviors and sleep bruxism commonly lead to sinus pain. Understanding that the nerve (trigeminal) connecting to many of the muscles in the face and the TMJ also conveys information from the sinus.

As a result, TMD therapy that reduces muscle problems can help provide relief of the sinus symptoms. You can also try the following to help relax your tense, overworked muscles to find relief from sinus pain:

- Jaw muscle exercises
- Jaw conditioning
- Massage
- Bite plates
- Injection therapy

The next time you are experiencing sinus complications, and traditional medications for sinus issues are not helping you might want to re-examine your jaw--that could have been the culprit all along.

Ear Pain

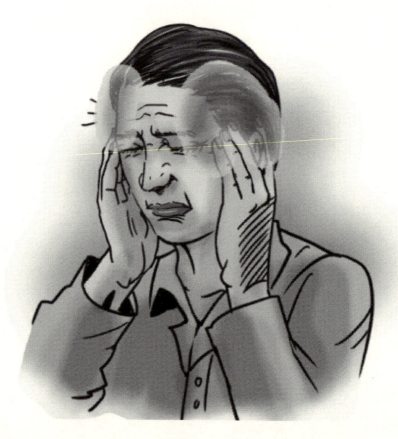

Yes, your ears can also experience aches and pains when you suffer from TMD. Other than when you were a child, you may not have experienced pain in your ears. Or, if you did, you simply brushed it off as a mild irritation.

However, ear problems are also linked with TMJ disorders. During the growth and development of the structures of your ear, the temporomandibular joint and the jaw muscles originate from similar cells—this means they share the same nerve pathways that can influence muscle tone and performance.

The most common cause of unexplained ear pain in an adult is temporomandibular joint disorder (TMD). The temporomandibular joint (TMJ) is located extremely close to the ear canal and middle ear. The muscles that surround the TMJ, and the fascia and ligaments that hold the bones in place are intricately connected with the ear and nerves that supports the ear.

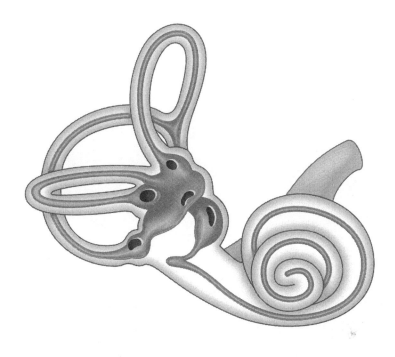

Pain frequently persists for several weeks, and may even come and go. Often the ear pain can get worse at night or in the morning. If treatment for the ear has not resolved your symptoms, then TMD might be a culprit for your suffering.

The muscle that runs along the length of the Eustachian tube (regulates ear pressure) is the same nerve that serves the jaw muscles. As a result, the TMJ can directly influence ear pain because of the changes in the way the Eustachian tube affects the ear. So, remember, ear pain is not always just a mild irritation—it might be more serious than you think.

Often after visiting your primary care physician, or an ENT, you may be diagnosed with Eustachian tube dysfunction (ETD). This diagnosis is given because the doctor might not be sure of the exact problem of the ear. If this is the case, consider getting your temporomandibular joint (TMJ) evaluated as a possible culprit.

Facial Pain

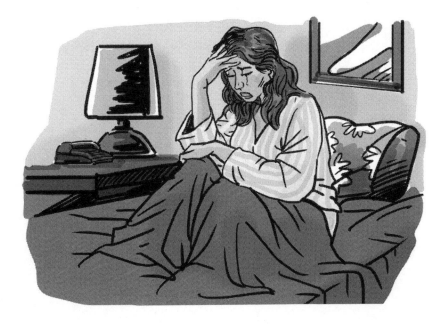

Problems involving facial pain can include temporomandibular joint (TMJ) discomfort, muscle spasms in the head, neck and jaw, cluster or frequent headaches, or pain with the teeth, face or jaw. If you have an unstable bite, missing teeth or poorly aligned teeth, you can experience pain and discomfort.

This is because your muscles are working harder than normal to bring your teeth together, which causes strain. Pain can even be a symptom of grinding or clenching your teeth (bruxism) and/or trauma to the head and neck.

With TMD, many patients experience facial pain, which can include pain or tenderness in the face, jaw joint area, neck and shoulders. And, as previously stated, facial pain can also include pain or tenderness in or around the ear when you chew, speak, or open your mouth wide.

In order to relieve facial pain, it is important to seek proper treatment for TMD, which can be overlooked when facial pain is being examined.

As a disorder that can wear many different hats, it is important to seek proper diagnosis and treatment planning from your dentist. Visiting your dentist will help in generating a diagnosis and determining if it is related to the temporomandibular joint or elsewhere.

Pain in Children and Teens

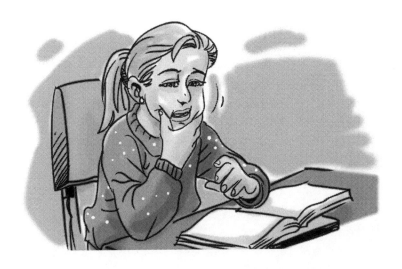

"The hardest part about being a parent is watching your children go through something really tough and not being able to fix it for them. All I am doing is all I can do..."

– Unknown Author

TMD, craniofacial and headache pain can also occur in children and teenagers. According to the American Academy of Pediatric Dentistry (AAPD), there is a rising concern about the presence of TMD, craniofacial pain and headaches among children and teens.

As you already know, the temporomandibular joint (TMJ) is the most complex joint in the human body. It consists of three major parts, including the lower jawbone, the pit of the temporal bone, and the associated connective tissue. The TMJ connects the lower jaw to the bone on the side of the head, which you can feel when placing your fingers in front of your ears and opening your mouth (Go ahead. Try it).

While almost everyone can experience soreness or tightness in their jaw from time to time, it can be a cause for concern in children and teens. Symptoms can sometimes go away after a few days, but it is best to seek diagnosis and treatment before further complication arises--especially if the soreness lasts for a few weeks. TMD can affect anyone, even children, but studies have shown it is much more common among teens, especially girls.

The TMJ begins to develop just six to seven weeks after conception. And the main components of the TMJ develop at a significant rate during a child's first 10 years of life. For this reason, injury to the jaw could impede or alter development if TMD is diagnosed.

While the TMJ tends to develop at a slower pace between the ages of 10 and 20, the mandibular condyle can change significantly during this period. The muscles and tendons continue to grow and strengthen during the pre-teen and teen years, which makes treating TMD tricky as children and teens grow.

Some possible causes of TMD in children and teens might be from frequent clenching of the jaw or teeth grinding. A lot of times this grinding can occur when a child is asleep. In the past, it has been thought that stress in children can contribute to a sudden development of symptoms of TMD because it makes them clench or grind their teeth while tightening their jaw muscles. However, this isn't the case for children, but in adults.

While adults might experience teeth grinding as a side effect of stress, children are typically not stressed. Instead, an area that is often overlooked is that in children, teeth grinding can be associated with not breathing well at night. Stress was once thought to be the cause, but we can now see that teeth grinding is airway related, meaning it occurs as a way to try to wake the brain up when breathing pauses.

Evaluating and treating children, as well as teenagers, can be difficult at times, as it requires further expertise than usual because the joints, teeth and facial muscles are still developing.

If your child is complaining about more than just one symptom of TMD, it is important to seek further diagnosis and treatment planning. It is imperative that TMJ complications are addressed immediately to prevent further complications and so corrective steps can be taken to relieve symptoms while halting further progression.

Symptoms of TMD

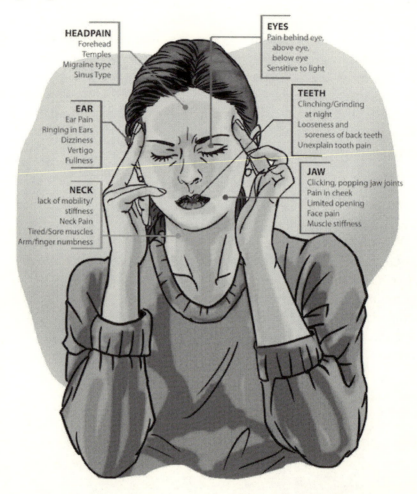

"Of pain you could wish only one thing: that it should stop. Nothing in the world was so bad as physical pain. In the face of pain there are no heroes."

- George Orwell, *1984*

TMD is usually easy to pinpoint due to the discomfort and pain that is experienced by the individual. You will notice pain in one or both sides of your face and it may be temporary but it may also last years if left untreated. You will begin to notice pain or tenderness in the jaw region, especially when you open your mouth to chew or speak.

Similarly, when eating you may notice clicking or popping sounds in the jaw joint which isn't always painful but can be quite annoying. Another unnerving symptom is jaws that may get stuck in the open or closed position.

Symptoms of TMD are characteristic of a number of other conditions, which makes diagnosis often very difficult. Some other symptoms that might mimic the characteristics of TMD include:

- Toothache
- Sinus infection
- Ear infection
- Facial neuralgias (nerve pain)
- Myofascial pain
- Headaches
- Unexplained ear ache

If pain in the jaw area is being experienced, tests will often be recommended to rule out or confirm the presence of any conditions, including TMD. All of these symptoms are concerning and can be very painful.

However, symptoms of TMD can also be misdiagnosed or connected to other conditions, such as fibromyalgia, vertigo, and tinnitus. But don't just take our word for it, see for yourself:

The TMD Connection

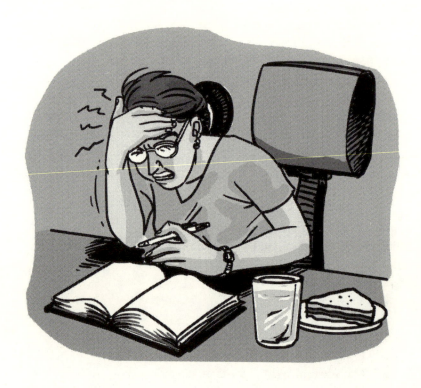

"Do not undervalue the headache. While it is at its sharpest it seems a bad investment; but when relief begins, the unexpired remainder is worth $4 a minute."

– Mark Twain

Many patients suffering from TMJ problems might also suffer from fibromyalgia. Unfortunately, many doctors don't recognize TMD or fibromyalgia or fail to see the connection of these two pain conditions. Fibromyalgia almost always intensifies the painful symptoms of TMD. Each disorder makes the other far worse than they would be on their own.

When one or both temporomandibular joints are affected, the pain of fibromyalgia in the neck and upper back are greatly magnified. Both TMD and fibromyalgia produce similar painful symptoms in the muscles of the neck, shoulders, back, face and head.

Unfortunately, many doctors who effectively treat fibromyalgia do not understand or recognize TMD and vice versa. Additionally, many patients who suffer from TMD have often been misdiagnosed as having fibromyalgia. For this reason, it is important to find proper diagnosis and treatment planning.

Finding Balance between Vertigo and TMD

Oh no, the world around you is spinning—or is it? It really isn't spinning, but you are definitely feeling dizzy, which is commonly called vertigo. While dizziness and vertigo are not serious, they will typically get better on their own. However, vertigo can also be a symptom of complications with TMD.

Temporomandibular joint disorder (TMD) can be a "great impostor," which causes postural imbalance that leads to a dizzying sensation of a person's surroundings.

Vertigo is a feeling that you are spinning or moving, while you are really standing in one place. So, what is the connection between vertigo and TMD? The connection begins with balance. It comes from the brain and integrates information from two main sources: 60% from the vestibular system in the inner ears and the other 40% from visual information.

It can also come from the "proprioception" information from stretch receptors of muscles and joints. This means it occurs at a subconscious level. It is a sense or feeling in your limbs or muscles that might be triggered by a condition elsewhere in the body, such as your ear.

In each inner ear, there is a structure that has three half-circles in three planes—superior, horizontal and posterior. These bony canals have fluid filled inner sacs where the sensing is accomplished by the movement of this fluid against hair like organs.

Each canal is oriented in such a way that the fluid moves when we move our head up and down, turn our head side to side, and when we tilt our head side to side over our shoulders.

The information from these balance organs has to integrate with the information from what we see and what we sense in our muscles and joints to give us balance. Your balance organ lies within the inner ear, which is housed in the petrous portion of the temporal bone.

If you put your little finger inside the ear canal and move your jaw by opening and closing, you can feel the movement of the mandible and realize how close it is to the inner ear (Go ahead and find it--we can wait).

If the mandible is poorly aligned with the upper jaw, then there are excessive pressures in the joint that is transmitted to the socket. In return, this can move the temporal bone just enough to move the balance organ—housed inside the ear—to be moved out of position as well.

Through neuromuscular treatment and oral appliance therapy, you can find relief from TMD and vertigo, as it helps to align the jaw properly.

Connecting TMD and Tinnitus

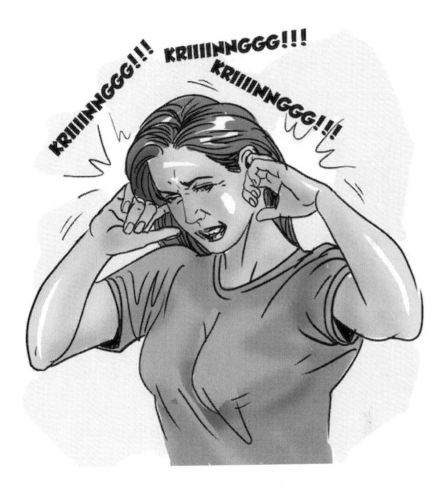

I am going slightly deaf in my right ear. It's tinnitus... something like that.
- Louis Tomlinson

Another connection with TMD might be Tinnitus, which is often referred to as "ringing of the ears," and can be one of the less common symptoms of TMJ disorders. Many patients suffering from temporomandibular joint disorder (TMD) with coexisting tinnitus find that TMD therapy often helps to improve or resolve their tinnitus in conjunction with their TMD symptoms.

There is a close relationship between certain problems with the TMJ and tinnitus. Some scientific studies show people with TMJ problems are more likely to suffer from tinnitus, while some individuals who have sustained an injury to their neck may also suffer from tinnitus. If you suffer from TMD or neck problems, you may find that you can alter the intensity of tinnitus by moving your mouth, jaw, face and neck.

Well that's interesting--tell me more! The chewing muscles are near some of the muscles that insert into the middle ear. This, in return, may have an effect on hearing, which promotes tinnitus. There is also a direct connection between the ligaments that attach to the jaw and one of the hearing bones that sits in the middle ear.

Through the nerve supply from the TMJ, a connection has been shown with the parts of the brain that are involved with both hearing and the interpretation of sound. The general discomfort associated with TMJ problems can also aggravate any pre-existing tinnitus. A variety of treatment options are currently available to help improve TMD symptoms, as well as symptoms of tinnitus.

Headaches and Migraines

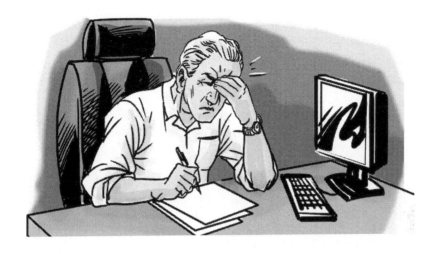

"His headache was still sitting over his right eye as if it had been nailed there."

— Ian Fleming, Moonraker

You've felt it before--that nagging, throbbing pain. Ouch! Headaches may often seem like a common occurrence for most people. However, it is important to understand that your headache can be more than just a common ache.

You might suffer from a headache or a migraine, but what you may not realize is the underlying cause to your pain might be related to your temporomandibular joint (TMJ). Let's take a closer look:

It is important for dentists to provide improved diagnosis and treatment options for those suffering from headaches, or worse, migraines. In order to alleviate your ache, it is important to reduce the number of risk factors present. Some common causal factors might include:

- Supporting your bite
- Improving sleeping habits
- Avoiding certain smells
- Drinking less or eliminating alcohol use
- Increasing exercise and losing weight
- Controlling teeth grinding
- Avoiding yeast and preservatives in food
- Improving posture

Depending on the cause of your migraine, a proper treatment plan will be created. From practicing preventive measures to managing contributing factors such as teeth grinding and a bad bite, dentists maintain the ability to successfully treat your ailments.

So say "Good-Bye" to migraines and hello to pain-free days.

Jaw Pain and Clicking

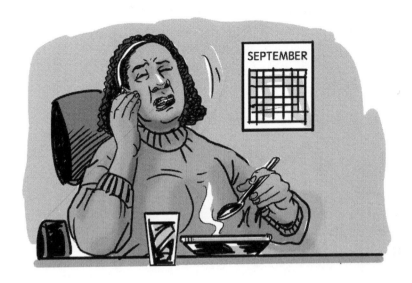

"To hurt is as human as to breathe."

- *J. K. ROWLING, The Tales of Beedle the Bard*

"Snap", "Crackle", and "Pop" should only be coming from your cereal, not your jaw. According to the National Institute of Craniofacial Research (NICR), TMJ complications affect more than 10 million people and it occurs more commonly in women than men. The sound of your jaw clicking can be a temporary annoyance or it can be a sign of TMD.

When we yawn, talk and chew food, we are using our temporomandibular joint (TMJ). Facial muscles attached to this joint control these movements. And a soft cartilage disc within the joint socket absorbs a massive amount of pressure so that no single motion does any damage.

But what happens when damage is done due to an injury or trauma, such as dislocation or a displaced disc? For most people, symptoms of TMD are mild and often disappear on their own, but for others, the pain can be persistent and debilitating.

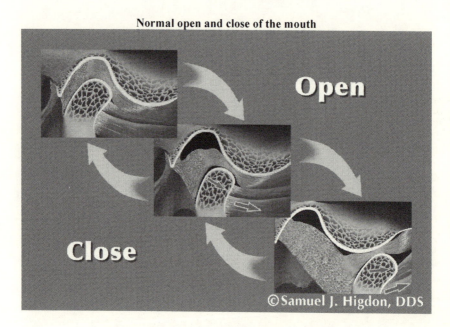

Normal open and close of the mouth

There are currently two types of jaw clicking or popping we can examine before any conclusions are made. One form of popping is when a person's mouth is at its widest--yawning.

This type of popping is more of a subluxation where the lower jawbone passes over a ridge in the upper jawbone. It is often a normal occurrence that is caused by just a hyperextended lower jaw. So, when you yawn next and a "popping" or "clicking" sound occurs, don't freak out just yet.

Next is the type of clicking or popping we need to be concerned about. This second type of clicking involves the displacement of the cartilage-like disc inside the joint. When you are closing your mouth, this popping typically occurs quietly.

The disc slips forward, in front of the lower jawbone. When you go to open your mouth again, a louder pop or crack will typically happen when the disc attempts to reposition itself onto the condyle of the lower jaw.

Opening the mouth with a pop

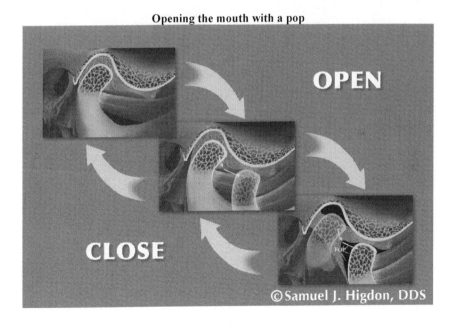

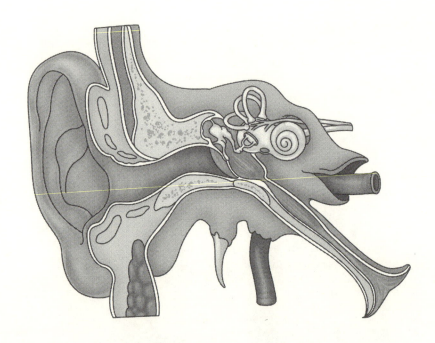

It can be bothersome to many people while eating or talking, and even painful. If you hear that snap, crackle and pop, and it isn't your cereal, you need to visit a specialist or dentist for further treatment.

You might also experience pain in the ear and joint if you clench your teeth. Clenching can occur either at night or during the day, or even both. The trouble with teeth clenching or grinding is that you might not realize it is occurring.

A helpful tip is if you catch yourself clenching, try to relax the jaw and maintain a lips together, teeth separated position—it might just make all the difference.

Misdiagnosing Fibromyalgia

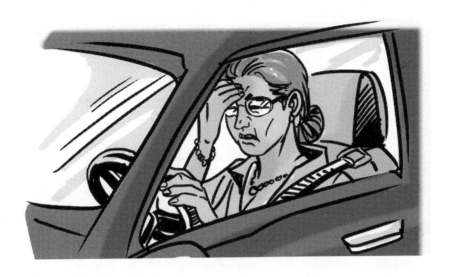

"Pain is such an uncomfortable feeling that even a tiny amount of it is enough to ruin every enjoyment."

– Will Rogers

To begin, what is fibromyalgia? Well, fibromyalgia is a chronic pain condition that can often lead to exhaustion with no known cause. That doesn't sound appealing, does it? No, it doesn't.

Imagine completing your daily tasks, but all of a sudden getting hit with an almost instant wave of exhaustion and pain--that is fibromyalgia. And, while it is not fatal, the pain can be excruciating. You might even find yourself visiting the emergency room or doctor after doctor to no avail—that in and of itself can be exhausting, too.

When fibromyalgia is diagnosed and treated properly, most people have a significant reduction in symptoms and a much better quality of life. However, diagnosing fibromyalgia is often difficult and symptoms can mimic other conditions, such as TMD.

With that being said, it is important to not only seek proper treatment, but proper diagnosis as well. To get a better understanding of this connection, we must look at the system overlap.

As mentioned previously, the main symptom of fibromyalgia is widespread pain. You can have pain on the right side, left side, or both sides of the body. It can also be above and below the waist—either way, it is extremely painful. The pain can even occur in only one or two places in the body, especially the neck and shoulders.

Diagnosing fibromyalgia can be tricky because it isn't the only condition with widespread pain. In addition to pain, another symptom of fibromyalgia is chronic fatigue. However, just like pain, patients with other conditions also have chronic fatigue, which makes the diagnosis even harder.

Pain and fatigue, as well as other symptoms of fibromyalgia, might be present in patients with other conditions, including the following:

- Thinking and memory problems
- Headaches
- Sensitivity to temperature, light, and noise
- Irritable bowel syndrome
- TMJ Disorder
- Morning stiffness
- Numbing or tingling of the extremities
- Sleep disturbances
- Urinary problems

Any combination of these symptoms can also suggest the presence of other illnesses, which makes proper diagnosis important.

Causes of TMD

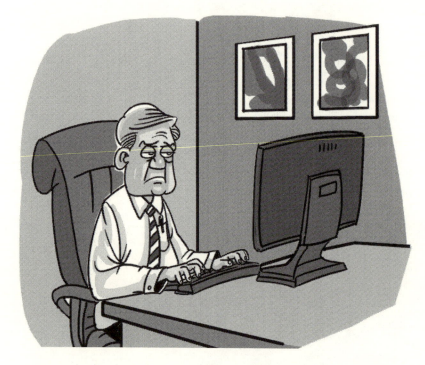

"The trouble with chronic pain is that it is so easy to become accustomed to it, both mentally and physically. At first it's absolutely agonizing; it's the only thing you think about, like a rock in your shoe that rubs your foot raw with every step. Then the constant rubbing, the pain and the limp all become part of the status quo, the occasional stabbing pain just a reminder. You are so set to endure, hunched against it - and when it starts to ease, you don't really notice, until the absence washes over you like a balm."

- Robert J. Wiersema, an Author and Writer

There are a wide variety of TMD causes, and they will vary from person-to-person depending on the situation. In most cases, any injury involving your jaw, jaw joint, or the muscles in your neck can contribute to TMD such as whiplash or a heavy blow to the face.

In other cases, issues involving grinding or clenching your teeth can be a huge factor. This creates a lot of stress for the jaw, which could cause you to experience pain. In more serious cases, there could be arthritis forming in the joint or a possible movement of soft cushion between the ball and socket. All of these situations can lead to a diagnosis of TMD.

When you are at risk, it increases your likelihood of getting a disease or condition. It is possible to develop TMD with or without the risk factors listed below. However, if you have a number of the risk factors listed, it is important to ask your dentist what you might be able to do to reduce your risk. Some causes or risk factors of TMD might include:

- **Stress** - If you are under a lot of stress in your life, you may have an increased risk of TMD. Some of the stress-related habits that may increase your risk of TMD are:
    - Habitually clenching and unclenching your jaw.
    - Grinding your teeth during the day and/or not breathing as a result of grinding.
    - Constantly chewing things, such as gum or ice.

- **Medical Conditions** - There are various medical conditions that can also increase your risk of TMD, including:
    - Misaligned teeth or bite
    - Jaw or facial deformities
    - Arthritic conditions
    - History of jaw or facial injuries

- **Gender** - Both men and women may suffer from TMD, but women account for 90 percent of those that seek treatment. Research continues to determine a possible connection between hormones and TMD, indicating that sometimes men and women process pain signals differently. However, there is no evidence to prove this claim quite yet.

- **Age** - Age can also play a factor in a person's risk for developing TMD. Individuals with TMD are most likely to be between the ages of 30 and 50 years of age. This does not always mean a person will develop TMD, but they are more likely.

- **Injury** - Trauma or injury to the jaw area can translate to long-term issues. TMD may develop if an injury causes dislocation of the jaw joint or movement of the disc and if muscles in opening and closing the jaw are weakened or strained, in addition to other complicating jaw conditions.

- **Other** – TMD can also be caused by a variety of other issues. For example, a person can develop TMD as the result of a sleep-breathing disorder or medication side effects.

While some cases of TMD cannot be cured, there are treatment options available to help prevent it from worsening and increasing pain. The underlying cause of TMD does not need to be known to provide quality care for a patient diagnosed with TMD.

With a proper understanding of what may be triggering your pain and controlling such factors, treatment success can be achieved.

Treatment Options for TMD

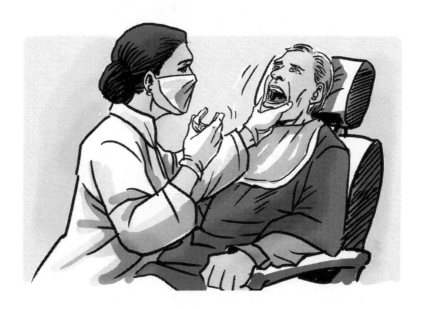

"Numbing the pain for a while will make it worse when you finally feel it."

- J.K. Rowling, *Harry Potter and the Goblet of Fire*

Temporomandibular joint disorders (TMD) are complex musculoskeletal health complications that impact neurological pain in the face. For many TMD sufferers, symptoms experienced can be difficult to manage.

When you suffer from jaw pain, it is important to become familiar with the risks faced and how you can sometimes manage by using home remedies. And, often, you might even ask, "Well, what else can I do to find relief?"

As we've mentioned several times already, when you experience pain, whether it is in the mouth or other parts of the body, it can be uncomfortable and interrupt your daily schedule. If you suffer from temporomandibular joint disorder (TMD), you don't have to simply "put up with" pain in the jaw. With help from your dentist's office, you can get the help you need to live with TMD without experiencing pain and discomfort.

Since the teeth, jaw joints, and muscles can all be involved, treatment for TMD varies from person to person. Typically, treatment will involve several phases. The first goal is to relieve the muscle spasm and pain. Next, your dentist must correct the way the teeth fit together. This device (known as an orthotic, or "splint") is worn over the teeth during the daytime until the bite is stabilized.

Permanent correction may involve the options below, but this is only performed once the splint has been worn and symptoms resolve. And if you're not able to go without the appliance, resulting in symptoms returning, then establishing your bite based on the splint position can be done with the following methods:

- Selective reshaping of the teeth
- Building crowns on the teeth
- Orthodontics
- A permanent appliance to lay over the teeth

If the jaw joint itself is damaged, it must be specifically treated. Though infrequent, surgery is sometimes required to correct a damaged joint.

Blindly making changes without trying a position can often lead to more symptoms. This is because it is like shooting in the dark with no end goal in sight.

Say Yes to Hot and Cold Packs

So, are hot and cold packs effective in providing relief from pain? The answer is yes. While hot and cold packs do not treat symptoms of TMD, they will work to help alleviate the aches and pains a person might be experiencing. Hot and cold packs should be rotated every 20 minutes to ensure the best accuracy and pain relief.

It might be recommended to place a cold pack to the side of the lower jaw (near the TMJ) for 10-20 minutes. And, after the cold pack is used, it is important to perform recommended stretches and/or exercises to help in the process and keep the TMJ from remaining stiff.

Next, apply a hot pack or warm towel to the joint. This routine should be repeated a few times each day to help alleviate some of the pain and stiffness of the TMJ.

Moist Heat Stretches

This form of TMD relief doesn't require much time on your part, but it can make all the difference. Go ahead and give it a try— you'll thank us in the end (we'll wait).

Whether you use a warm, moist towel at the sink, or spend a little extra time in a warm shower, moist heat stretches are important for relief. Start by spending some extra time in the shower. You can do this by letting the water flow over your painful areas. Feels good, doesn't it?

Next, soak a washcloth with warm water in your shower. As you are standing, place the warm washcloth on your jaw joint and open for about five seconds. Do this for a few minutes every time you shower.

If you forget to do moist heat stretches in the shower, try following the second photo (on the next page) by using a warm cloth at the sink.

In shower exercises or stretches

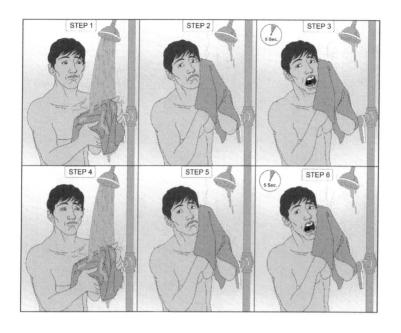

Out of shower exercises or stretches

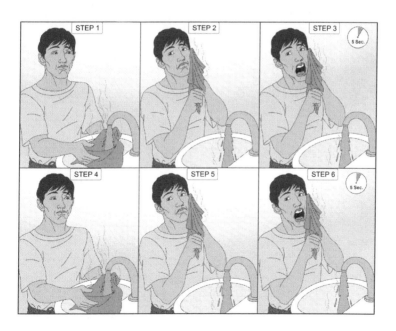

Oral Appliance Therapy

While hot or cold packs can help to alleviate pain and stiffness periodically, it is important to remember that this should not be the only form of treatment patients seek. Through the availability of oral appliance therapy, which helps to treat TMD symptoms, complex conditions can be successfully managed and treated.

Oral appliances may help reduce tension on the jaw muscles and the joint. Permanent changes in the bite through extensive crown or bridgework and orthodontics have not been proven to be effective in some cases and may worsen TMD symptoms.

If a contributing factor is teeth grinding or clenching, a splint or night guard can be worn while sleeping. Clenching and grinding cannot be stopped, but the oral appliance will help prevent tooth-to-tooth wear. Oral appliances can also help reduce the over working of muscles, which minimizes pain. The goal is that TMD symptoms will be reduced as the affected area experiences a period of reduced irritation and use.

In other instances, if the severity of the TMD condition is much more intrusive and painful, more invasive treatment options might be required. However, special care must be taken before deciding to undergo any invasive solution. Surgical treatments are often irreversible and remain controversial, as they have not been proven effective by any studies or research.

Take a look at the images on the next page—these are just two examples of oral appliances. The top photo is of an anterior deprogrammer splint worn at night, which helps to find comfortable joint position, and helps prevent the forces from clenching and bruxism (teeth grinding) to affect the teeth, joints and muscles. The bottom image is of a lower reposition appliance worn during the day, which is used to reposition the mandible (jaw) in a forward position—this helps in realigning your jaws.

Anterior Deprogrammer Splint Worn at Night

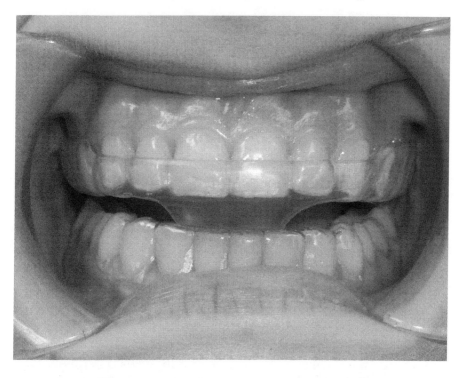

Lower Reposition Appliance Worn During the Day

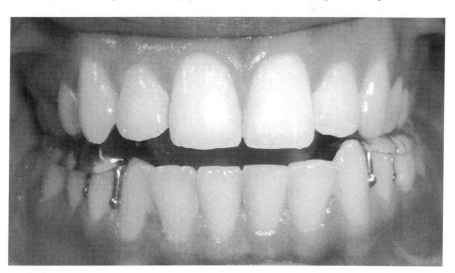

Physical Therapy

A doctor or physical therapist may recommend stretches that can help reduce tension in the jaw. Perform prescribed exercises as directed to stretch the muscles of the jaw and relieve unnecessary muscle tension. The use of physical therapy includes learning and practicing techniques for regaining normal jaw movement again.

The focus of physical therapy for TMD is relaxation, stretching and releasing tight muscles and scar tissue--it is especially important in recovery from TMJ surgery, and helping to minimize scar tissue formation and muscle tightness. Physical therapy techniques may include the following:

- Jaw exercises to strengthen muscles and improve flexibility and range of motion.
- Dry needling to resolve trigger points in muscles.
- Heat therapy to improve blood circulation in the jaw.
- Ice therapy to reduce swelling and relieve pain.
- Massage to relieve overall muscle tension.
- Training to improve posture and correct jaw alignment.
- Transcutaneous electrical nerve stimulation (TENS), which utilizes a mild electrical current to the skin over the jaw joint to help relax muscles, improve blood circulation and relieve pain.

After treatment with physical therapy it is important to rest the jaw, try to control habits that might cause jaw pain and avoid chewing foods that will cause stress to the TMJ. In doing so, you can further extend the relief from pain and improve overall jaw function.

Medications. When experiencing pain caused by TMD, some over-the-counter medications can help dull the pain of your spasms. These OTC drugs can help you cope with pain from spasms if other techniques are not working. However, it is always important to consult your dentist before doing so.

Over-the-counter pain relievers such as ibuprofen, acetaminophen, and naproxen can minimize the experience of pain and reduce inflammation. A doctor may also prescribe stronger pain medications for pain relief. Prescription muscle relaxants may aid patients who grind their teeth by relaxing the muscles of the jaw. Low doses of antidepressants have also been found to reduce pain.

Create a Self-Treatment Schedule. This may sound strange, but by creating a self-treatment schedule we can establish a successful way to improve your condition.

For example, a person's schedule should include regularly performing exercises as recommended by your dentist to improve your symptoms of TMD. Contact your dentist's office today to learn more about how to manage your symptoms at home.

Reduce Tension and Stress. People who suffer from TMD should also undertake daily activities to help reduce tension and stress. Try yoga, meditation, or breathing exercises to release stress and tightness in the muscles of the face, neck, shoulders and back. By relieving stress, you can further help in eliminating the pains experienced with TMD.

This might seem silly, but deep breathing can help to alleviate your stress, which can, in turn, help to reduce your TMJ spasms. Try sitting with your feet on the floor and your hand on your stomach.

Breathe in deeply through your nose and then exhale, pushing gently on your stomach with your hand—this can help you breathe deeper. You might also want to try medication or relaxation training to further relieve stress, which can also help to relieve TMJ spasms.

Avoid high-tension jaw movement: Moving the jaw with excessive force can strain the joint and the muscles that open and close the mouth, and hamper treatments aimed at reducing the pain. Yawning and chewing should be kept to a minimum. Singing or yelling should also be avoided.

Proper posture while on the phone or at a computer should be maintained. Avoid clenching the jaw. Practice keeping your teeth apart by gently placing your tongue on the roof of your mouth, behind your upper front teeth, with your teeth slightly separated.

Practicing stress reduction techniques to relax muscle tension in the jaw can help alleviate some of the pain and swelling associated with TMD.

Maintain a Good Posture. Maintaining good posture at work, while driving, at home, and during recreational activities helps to relieve muscle and joint tension in the jaw, neck, back and head.

You should also avoid holding the phone between your shoulder and ear. Instead, try to hold the phone with a hand to your ear, or by using a headset to avoid crunching the muscles of the neck and shoulder—causing unnecessary strain.

Join a Support Group. It may sound strange, but there are support groups out there for those suffering from TMD. For example, the TMJ Association helps to educate patients on how to minimize the effect of painful and disabling symptoms.

They also update members on the latest research and news in TMD studies, and offers a supportive and understanding community to ask questions and share experiences.

Sometimes hearing what others are doing to improve their symptoms is all you might need to find relief from your own symptoms.

Surgery. The use of surgery for TMD is rarely needed. However, there are a small percentage of patients who do not see improvement from conservative treatment, and must consult an oral and maxillofacial surgeon.

With several surgeries available, it is important to find the best treatment option for relief from your pain.

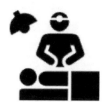

The three surgery options available for the treatment of TMD include the following:

- **Arthrocentesis** - This surgery option is used if you have no major history of TMD but your jaws are locked. It is a minor procedure performed in oral surgery where you will receive anesthesia, then needles will be inserted into the joint and washed out.

- **Arthroscopy** - This surgery is performed with an arthroscope, which is a special tool with a lens and light on it. You will receive general anesthesia and then a small cut will be made in front of the ear and the tool inserted.

  The tool is hooked up to a video screen in order to examine the joint and the area around it. Inflamed tissue may be removed or the disc may be realigned. This surgery is known to be minimally invasive, leaves a smaller scar, has fewer complications and requires a shorter recovery time than a major operation.

- **Open-Joint Surgery** - Depending on the cause of your TMD, arthroscopy may not be possible. If that is the case, it would mean you might need open-joint surgery. This type of surgery might be needed if the bony structure in your jaw joint are wearing down, you have tumors in or around the joint, and your joint is scarred or full of bone chips.

  Recovery time after open-joint surgery will be needed and there is a greater chance of scarring and nerve injury.

Receiving proper diagnosis is vital in preparing for proper treatment. Trying conservative non-surgical options should always be attempted before considering surgery in some cases. When experiencing pain, it is important to not ignore pain or it could worsen.

Watch What You Eat

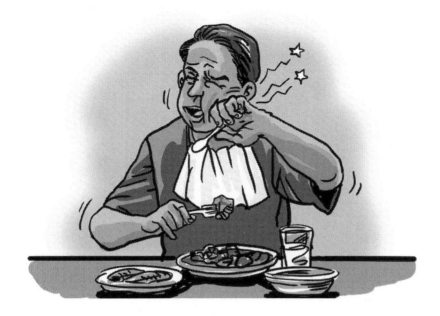

"People who love to eat are always the best people."

- Julia Child

Without proper nutrition you increase the risk of either gaining or losing weight, or suffering from nutritional deficiencies due to the pain caused by TMD. And through this, it can lead to other health problems. When it comes to maintaining your health and diet, remember to eat fruits, vegetables, starches, protein and dairy, but be mindful of your TMD as you do so.

Many people who suffer from TMD tend to struggle with determining what to eat in order to maintain a proper weight and ensure adequate protein, vitamin and mineral status. Your food choices will vary depending on the amount of pain you experience and your ability to open your mouth, chew and swallow.

For those who are able to adequately open their mouths and have minimal pain, a soft or easy to chew diet will work well. A soft diet is defined as food that requires minimal chewing, including:

- **Dairy/Dairy Alternatives:** Smooth yogurt, soft cheeses, milk, custard, puddings, and soymilk.
- **Grains:** Soft bread, corn bread, muffins without seeds or nuts, soft tortillas, pancakes, and quinoa.
- **Fruits:** Canned fruits, bananas, ripe melon, baked apples, fruit juice, and fruit smoothies.
- **Vegetables:** Cooked carrots, squash, zucchini, spinach, kale or other greens, avocados, green beans, and cooked pumpkin.
- **Protein Foods:** Soft-cooked chicken or turkey with gravy, meatloaf, fish, deli meats, meatballs, tuna, refried beans, and smooth nut butters.
- **Soups:** Cream-based soups, tomato soup, and broth-based soups.
- **Desserts:** Soft cakes, cobblers and pies, frozen yogurt, sherbet, milkshakes and puddings.

If you are unable to tolerate a soft diet, a pureed diet may be a better option for you. Some examples of foods that can be included in a pureed diet are:

- **Dairy/Dairy Alternatives:** Smooth yogurt, soft cheeses, milk, custard, puddings, and soymilk.
- **Grains:** Bread that has been soaked into a dissolvable consistency, pureed pasta, hot cereals, grits, and mashed potatoes.
- **Fruits:** Applesauce, mashed ripe bananas, fruit juice, and seedless jam/jelly.
- **Vegetables:** Mashed white or sweet potatoes, pureed carrots, beets, beans, peas, creamed corn and hummus.
- **Protein Foods:** Pureed meats, pureed/scrambled eggs, crust-less quiche, egg custards, and yogurt-based smoothies.
- **Soups:** Soups that are smooth or that have been put through the blender.
- **Desserts:** Puddings, custards, dessert soups, gelatin, and fondue.

Keeping a list of foods you can eat, and foods not to eat, is a good place to start in ensuring you are eating the right foods to better protect your jaw. On the next page you will find a list of good food choices if you suffer from temporomandibular joint disorder (TMD).

However, it is still important to consult your doctor or dentist to learn more about proper foods to eat.

Food Choices for TMD Sufferers

For those who are able to adequately open their mouths and have minimal pain, a soft or easy to chew diet will work well. A soft diet is defined as food that requires minimal chewing, including:

Dairy/Dairy Alternatives: Smooth yogurt, soft cheeses, milk, custard, puddings, and soy milk.

Fruits: Canned fruits, bananas, ripe melon, baked apples, fruit juice, and fruit smoothies.

Grains: Soft bread, corn bread, muffins without seeds or nuts, soft tortillas, pancakes, and quinoa.

Vegetables: Cooked carrots, squash, zucchini, spinach, kale or other greens, avocados, green beans, and cooked pumpkin.

Protein Foods: Soft-cooked chicken or turkey with gravy, meatloaf, fish, deli meats, refried beans, and smooth nut butters.

Soups: Cream-based soups, tomato soup, and broth-based soups.

Desserts: Soft cakes, cobblers and pies, frozen yogurt, sherbet, milkshakes and puddings.

www.mpateldds.com

The Connection Between Pain and Sleep

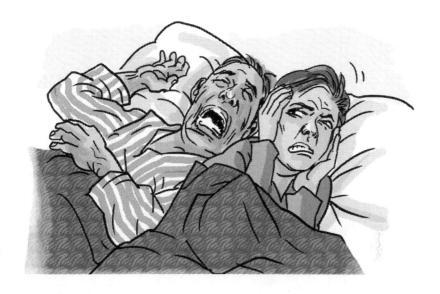

"Laugh and the world laughs with you, snore and you sleep alone."

– Anthony Burgess

First, before we dive into the connection between pain and sleep, let's look at the idea of sleep and just how important it is for us. We sleep every night (or at least we hope we get to). But have you ever wondered why we need to sleep? Even more so, why is good sleep so important?

A good night's sleep is one of the most important things for you in regards to your health. In fact, sleep is just as important as eating healthy and exercising! Nowadays people are sleeping less than they did in the past and sleep quality has decreased, too. The advancements in technology and our everyday lives are interfering with natural sleep patterns.

The way you feel while you are awake depends in part on what happens while you're sleeping. During sleep, your body is working to support healthy brain function and maintain your physical health, while, in children and teens; sleep also helps support growth and development.

The damage from sleep deficiency can occur instantly or it can take time to harm you. For instance, lack of sleep or quality sleep, can harm you by increasing your chances in being involved in a car crash, but it can further harm you over time when chronic health problems are involved.

Healthy Brain Function

We sleep to support healthy brain function because this is when your brain is able to prepare for the next day. During sleep, your brain is forming new pathways to help you learn and remember information. It has been shown that a good night's sleep improves learning no matter the subject. Sleep also helps you to pay attention, make decisions, and be creative.

And, if you are sleep deficient, you may have trouble with your emotions, as it has been linked to depression, suicide and risk-taking behavior. Children and teens that are not getting enough sleep may experience problems with:

- Getting along with others
- Feeling angry and impulsive
- Having mood swings,
- Feeling sad or depressed
- Exhibiting a lack of motivation.

A lack of sleep might also lead to problems paying attention and a negative effect on their grades.

Physical Health

Sleep is important for your physical health because it is involved in healing and repairing of your heart and blood vessels. With ongoing sleep deficiency, people can experience an increased risk of heart disease, kidney disease, high blood pressure, diabetes, and stroke. A lack of sleep can also increase the risk of obesity.

Our immune system relies on sleep to stay healthy because this is the system that defends the body against foreign or harmful substances. Ongoing sleep deficiency can change the way in which the immune system responds.

A Lack of Sleep and Increased Pain

The amount of pain related to sleep loss is astounding. Millions of Americans are experiencing a lack of sleep due to pain, which can be avoided with proper care. In the 2015 "Sleep in America Poll", about 21 percent of Americans experience chronic pain, while 36 percent has had acute pain in the past week.

If you combine those numbers with the majority of the nation's adult population (57 percent), it leaves about 43 percent who report being pain-free--now that is not a high enough number. With so many people complaining of pain and a lack of sleep, why don't more people do something to fix their symptoms? It's because they don't always know what to do.

Pain is often a combination of stress and poor health, as it correlates to shorter sleep durations and worsens the quality of sleep experienced. However, there are ways to resolve this issue.

By making sleep a priority, the sleep gap can narrow significantly. On average, according to the National Sleep Foundation, there's a 42-minute sleep debt for those with chronic pain and 14 minutes for those who have suffered from acute pain in the past week.

On the other hand, there is no overall sleep debt for those without pain. However, a significant number in this group do have sleep problems with about one in three saying they don't always, or don't often get enough sleep each night. These issues rise even higher in individuals who do have chronic or acute pain.

By making sleep a priority, it is linked to better sleep, even among those who complain of chronic or acute pain.

Case Studies

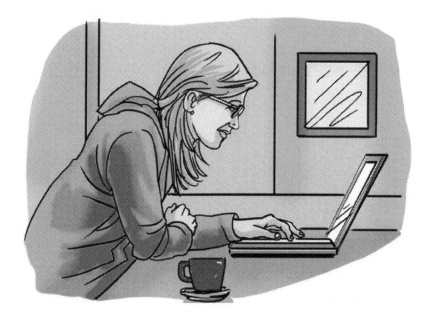

We understand that providing all of this information on TMD is one thing, but where's the proof? Relax—we've got that covered. To better showcase just how important TMD treatment is, as well as proper diagnosis from a qualified dentist, here are some case studies that properly showcase TMD treatment and how much of a difference it has made in their daily lives.

The Initial Examination

When a diagnosis is made, several things will need to be gathered at an initial exam. The most important part is the questionnaire that asks specific questions about:

- Various conditions and symptoms
- Severity, location and quality of pain
- Medication history
- What makes the pain worse or better
- Previous treatments and outcomes

Next will be an interview to get an understanding of symptoms followed by a clinical examination and necessary testing to assist in a diagnosis. This then allows for treatment recommendations.

As American poet, Edward Hodnett once said, "If you do not ask the right questions, you do not get the right answers. A question asked in the right way often points to its own answer. Asking questions is the A-B-C of diagnosis. Only the inquiring mind solves problems."

Case 1
Patient: Madison
Age: 18

Meet Madison, an 18-year-old female. Madison's chief complaints upon entering my office were jaw pain, limited mouth opening and facial pain. She had no known allergies and was currently on birth control medication. Her past medical history included prior orthodontic treatment, psychiatric care, sinus problems and tendency for ear infections. Additionally, Madison's current medical history included:

- Anxiety
- Asthma
- Chronic Pain
- Difficulty Sleeping
- Mood Disorder
- Nasal Allergies
- Wisdom Teeth extraction

A past surgical procedure she had was a Frenotomy (the removal of a frenulum, a small fold of tissue that prevents an organ in the body from moving too far) while her family history included high blood pressure, thyroid disorder and snoring (her father). It is important to note all past and current information. It is pertinent in establishing proper diagnosis and treatment planning—so don't leave any information out!

Without knowing your history, it could have negative consequences on your health. Moving on, Madison is a student who denies ever smoking and consumes about one drink with caffeine per day, while also performing regular exercise.

Symptoms: Madison's symptoms included the following:

- Frontal headaches (left side)
- Temporal headaches (left side)
- Jaw pain upon opening on the left

- Jaw pain while chewing on the left
- Jaw pain while at rest on the left
- Clenching teeth
- Burning tongue
- Ear congestion on the left
- Pain behind the ear (left side)
- Recurrent ear infections
- Lower back pain
- Upper back pain
- Neck pain
- Shoulder pain
- Swollen glands

Now that's a lot of symptoms for one person to be experiencing, isn't it? We thought so, too.

Treatment History: She has also received the following treatment from these doctors:

- Dr. EB; Specialty: Oral Surgeon; Treatment: wisdom teeth extraction
- Dr. PK; Specialty: TMJ – treatment for her limited mouth opening.
- Dr. JS; dentist – help with limited mouth opening and face pain

The difference between each of the doctors was that Dr. JS referred Madison to us for proper treatment--he knew we could offer the right solution.

History of Present Illness: Madison believes the cause of her pain or condition is from dental procedures. She states the pain or condition first occurred after her wisdom teeth extraction procedure on July 14, 2015, when on July 25th her jaw locked up while eating cereal.

She reports that pain is equally worse on both sides, and her headache spreads to the temple. Based on the numeric pain scale of 1-10, Madison complains of:

- Jaw pain is a level of 9
- Headaches are a 3
- Neck pain is a 2
- Facial pain is a 4, constant and lasting for weeks

Madison's pain is constant, lasting for weeks, and also experiences fatigue and throbbing.

Objective: Mild tenderness was reproduced upon palpation of the temporal tendon on the right, splenius capitis on the left, occipital bilaterally, buccinator insertion on the left, buccinator origin on the left, medial pterygoid on the left, deep masseter on the right, posterior joint space on the right, lateral TMJ capsule on the right, sternocleidomastoid on the left, stylomandibular ligament bilaterally and superficial masseter on the right.

Moderate tenderness was reproduced upon palpation of the styloid process on the right and superficial masseter on the left. Severe tenderness was elicited upon palpation of the deep masseter on the left, temporal tendon on the left, lateral TMJ capsule on the left and posterior joint space on the left. Clinical examination revealed the TM joints within normal limits.

Cranial Nerve II-XII Screening: Within normal limits. Cervical range of motion measurements indicated pain on flexion, pain on extension, pain on side bend (bilateral) and pain on rotation on both sides.

Mandibular Range of Motion Measurements: Maximum opening of 22 mm with pain, maximum protrusive of 2 mm, left lateral excursion of 6 mm, right lateral excursion of 8 mm, normal mandibular midline, normal maxillary midline and normal skeletal midlines. Normal opening is opening over 40mm and your jaw moving side to side (lateral) to be over 10mm and moving your jaw forward (protruding) being 8mm.

Oral Examination: Missing teeth 1,16,17,32, a 1 mm overbite, a 1 mm overjet, tongue level 2, grade 2 mallampati classification, biting on cotton rolls on both sides produced pain on left side, biting on a cotton roll on the left side produced pain on left side, application of Spray and Stretch improved maximum opening to 39 mm. Tomography reviewed and all is within normal limits. Mandibular fixed retainer.

Assessment: Working diagnosis is bilateral myalgia, capsulitis of the bilateral temporomandibular joint and limited mandibular range of motion. Wait, what? In other words, Madison had muscle pain on both sides of her face muscles, also her TMJ hurt when you touched it and she was not able to open wide.

Treatment Plan and Goals: After assessment, these included:

- Improve Myalgia (muscle pain)
- Improve Range of Motion
- Patient Education
- Reduce Adverse Joint Loading
- Reduce Pain

To accomplish these goals I recommended oral orthopedic appliance therapy to control jaw function and masticatory forces. They would also improve the biomechanics of the TM joint region and aid in improving TM joint symptoms. Medication regimen included Flexeril (a muscle relaxant) at night prn. Disp 30 tabs and recommended moist heat stretches. We also decided to control her nighttime grinding with a simple upper mouth guard.

At her two week follow up Madison was experiencing no pain and was able to open to 51mm, with side movements of 15mm. She was astatic that simply wearing a night guard resolved her issue. Her frustration was seeing multiple doctors that suggested her bite was limited because of her disc being out (only way to confirm that would be a MRI) and told that jaw surgery was the only way to resolve it.

Case 2
Patient: Mr. Chad
Age: 32

Meet Mr. Chad, a 32-year-old male. At his initial visit, Mr. Chad's complains included:

- Migraines
- Fatigue
- Morning head pain
- Teeth grinding
- Dizziness
- Jaw clicking
- Headaches
- Jaw locking
- Facial pain
- Neck pain
- Jaw pain
- Tooth pain

It was quite the list of complaints and I could sense the frustration he was experiencing. He was currently taking ½ an Ambien once every night to help with getting sleep. When he would not take it he found himself waking up in even more pain.

Past medical history for Mr. Chad was another long list, including:

- Acid Reflux
- Anxiety
- Chronic Fatigue
- Chronic Pain
- Depression
- Dizziness
- Insomnia
- Tendency for ear infections, tumors and wisdom teeth extraction

At that time, he was experiencing difficulty sleeping and fibromyalgia. As for past surgical procedures, Mr. Chad had a cyst removal over his right posterior maxillary area. And his family History included high blood pressure, a sleep disorder, and snoring (father).

Symptoms: Mr. Chad's lengthy list of symptoms included:

- Jaw pain upon opening on both sides
- Jaw pain while chewing on both sides
- Jaw pain while at rest on both sides
- Jaw clicking on both sides
- Jaw popping
- Jaw locks open
- Teeth grinding
- Clenching teeth
- Frequent snoring
- Pain in front of the ear
- Middle back pain
- Upper back pain
- Neck pain
- Shoulder pain
- Shoulder stiffness
- Swelling in the neck
- Tightness in throat
- Tingling in the hands or fingers

Treatment History: From 2015 to the present, Mr. Chad had multiple visits to various Urgent Care centers and multiple dental visits to various dentists in an attempt to get to the bottom of his tooth pain and jaw pain. He even had visits to two neurologists, an oral surgeon, physical therapist and a massage therapist. Mr. Chad found us off the Internet while doing research to figure out what he might have and whom he should visit.

History of Present Illness: Mr. Chad believes the cause of the pain or condition is from an injury, such as a motor vehicle accident or even a possible soccer injury--both are very plausible reasons. He states the pain or condition first occurred Sept 1,

2015, and when asked "Is there anything that makes your pain or discomfort worse?" he stated, "not stretching, not getting a massage, not getting dry needling, sleeping, and stress".

Regarding the question, "Is there anything that makes your pain or discomfort better?" Mr. Chad stated, "Massages, dry needling, stretching using a hardened racquet ball to rub on temporalis and masseter". He believes other information important to the pain or condition to be, "It keeps recurring and tightening. Never goes away".

Pain is reported as worse on the left side, headache spreads to the temple, and pain on a numeric pain scale of 0-10 includes:

1. Jaw pain is 5
2. Headaches are a 2
3. Neck pain is a 5
4. Facial pain is a 5 and constant

When having pain, Mr. Chad reports dizziness, nausea, sensitivity to noise and a throbbing feeling. His fatigue and pain has isolated him in his own home. Returning from work he would medicate himself and go to bed. Weekends were no different for him, but to deal with activities of daily living he would push through. He even made the move to live with his mom because he needed help.

Objective: Mild tenderness was reproduced upon palpation of the posterior joint space on the left, trapezius neck area bilaterally, middle temporalis on the right, and lateral TMJ capsule bilaterally. In his clinical examination, it was revealed that the temporomandibular joints were within normal limits.

Cranial nerve screening revealed a possible deficit in the following nerves: V - Division II and III on his right side. This was due to the wisdom teeth he had extracted that damaged his nerves. Cervical range of motion measurements indicated pain on flexion, pain on extension, pain on side bend (right side) and pain on rotation on the right.

Mandibular range of motion measurements revealed 60 mm opening without pain, maximum protrusive of 8 mm, left lateral excursion of 14 mm, right lateral excursion of 13 mm, 0 mm overbite and 0 mm overjet.

Oral examination revealed missing teeth 1,2,16,17,32, tongue level 2, grade 2 mallampati classification, dental crossbite on both sides of his back teeth, biting on a cotton roll on the left side produced pain on left side and biting on a cotton roll on the right side produced pain on left side. Mr. Chad presented with a Class III (protruded lower jaw) dental relationship. The mandibular dental midline was to the left by approximately 5 mm.

Assessment: Working diagnosis is arthritis/capsulitis of both temporomandibular joints and myalgia on both sides.

Treatment Plan and Goals: Treatment was directed toward improving myalgia, patient education, and reducing adverse joint loading. The treatment plan consists of oral orthopedic appliance therapy to control jaw function and masticatory forces. They would also improve the biomechanics of the TMJ region and aid in improving TM joint symptoms. Plan on insertion of a maxillary orthotic to help control the forces of parafunction during sleep.

Chad's history stated that stress made his symptoms worse, which often occurred when he awoke from sleep. Those are some strong statements that could suggest what he was doing while sleeping played a big role in his symptoms.

After looking over his examination findings we felt that it would be appropriate to control his nighttime forces with a bite guard. We set off to do just that.

After two weeks from the time we initially saw Chad, we delivered his device. Chad was excited and very optimistic that the nighttime guard would hopefully make a difference.

However, he was also a bit reserved since other dentists had made him guards with very little positive outcomes.

Where we differed from the previous dentists was the fact that when he slept his back teeth would not touch the guard just his front. The idea being that when back teeth make contact there is a tendency for you to clench more, generating more force.

At his two week follow up I was shocked to see him in the treatment room with a smile on his face like he just won the lottery! As I walked in he stood up and firmly shook my hand as he said, "thank you" multiple times. I was not sure for what but after questioning him on his past two weeks I quickly learned he was feeling 100 times better than the weeks prior to wearing his guard.

If you recall Chad's initial symptoms, he was no longer experiencing any morning head pain, nor jaw pain. Additionally, in the past two weeks he has not had a migraine, and he even felt like he has more energy.

He was not fatigued, and even started to walk and jog again whereas before he would go to bed once he got home from work because he was in pain and felt so drained. The unexplained toothache he was having was resolved and the dizziness he used to experience had also resolved. Mr. Chad could not believe that wearing the guard we fabricated made all the difference in the world.

It was the type of guard that made the difference, or the fact that he was now understanding what his triggers were that allowed us to better get to the root of his problems. Taking into account a patient's history can often point you down the right path for a proper treatment approach. Dentists strive to listen and allow our patients to talk. We can often guide you through the use of questions in order to get a better understanding of your health concerns.

Case 3

Patient Name: Gregory
Age: 49

Meet Gregory, a 49-year-old male. Gregory visited my office with the following complaints:

- Fatigue
- Headaches
- Morning head pain
- Jaw pain
- Jaw clicking
- Frequent heavy snoring
- Neck pain
- Difficulty concentrating and focusing because of pressurized feeling near his right jaw

Gregory reported allergic reactions to no known allergens. He was currently taking a variety of medications (it's a long list we don't need to share). Just know it was a lot to take in every day, so we wanted to find him a better solution.

Significant Medical History: In the past, Gregory suffered from the following: Anxiety, anemia, bleeding easily, chronic fatigue, chronic pain, depression, difficulty sleeping, neuralgia, psychiatric care, sinus problems, sleep apnea, tendency for ear infections, urinary disorders, wisdom teeth extraction and Seborrheic Dermatitis.

And, currently, Gregory expressed the following medical history: Anxiety, anemia, chronic fatigue, chronic pain, depression, difficulty sleeping, neuralgia, sinus problems, sleep apnea, urinary disorders and Seborrheic Dermatitis.

His past surgical procedures included an appendectomy, gallbladder, hernia repair, Jaw Joint, nasal, tonsillectomy and Hernia Removal/ Repair 1972, wisdom teeth extraction 1990's, straighten deviated septum April 1991, TMJ surgery April 1994, Tonsillectomy July 1996, Gallbladder removed April 2005, Appendectomy April 2007, Spinal Cord April 2007, TMJ Surgery September 2013. Additionally, his family history included cancer, heart disease, diabetes, high blood pressure, stroke, sleep disorder, snoring (father) and sleep apnea (father).

Symptoms of constant moderate generalized headaches (bilateral), constant moderate temporal headaches (right side), jaw pain upon opening on both sides, jaw pain while chewing on both sides, jaw pain while at rest on both sides, jaw clicking on both sides, jaw popping, jaw locks closed, jaw locks open, teeth grinding, clenching teeth, ear congestion, hearing loss, pain behind the ear, lower back pain, middle back pain, difficulty in swallowing, neck pain and scoliosis, pressure around and behind right ear causing concentration and focus problems.

Treatment History:

Dr. GL; Specialty: Oral surgeons; Treatment: jaw surgery on his right; Date: 4-1994
Dr. GB; Specialty: Oral surgeons: Treatment jaw surgery on his right; Date: 9-2013

History of Present Illness: Gregory stated the pain or condition first occurred mid January 1990. When asked, "Is there anything that makes your pain or discomfort worse?" he stated, "sleeping and not moving my jaw much. I'm worse in the morning."

He believes other information important to the pain or condition to be, "I was chewing on a hard candy and something felt like it ripped or tore in or near the jaw joint. It made an internal noise I could hear. For days afterwards, it sounded like a blood flowing sound from that area."

Gregory also stated a few years ago he had a steroid injection in his foot and the symptoms he was having in his jaw area and throat resolved for some time.

When discussing his pain, Gregory reported pain as worse on the right side, headache spreading to the temple, and very near the ear and jaw area too. On a numeric scale of 0-10, Gregory listed:

- Jaw pain is a level of 7
- Headaches are a 5
- Neck pain is a 3 and constant

When having pain, Gregory also reports fatigue and photophobia. With so much pain and discomfort, it is no wonder why Gregory continues to remain frustrated with his condition.

Initial Analysis: Mild tenderness was elicited upon palpation of the superficial masseter on the right, trapezius neck area on the right, temporal tendon on the left, posterior joint space bilaterally, anterior temporalis bilaterally, middle temporalis on the left and posterior temporalis bilaterally.

Moderate tenderness was elicited upon palpation of the lateral TMJ capsule bilaterally and middle temporalis on the right. Clinical examination revealed the TMJs were within normal limits and the cranial nerve II-XII screening was within normal limits. Cervical range of motion was within normal limits.

An interesting fact was the duration of his pain and two failed TMJ surgeries. Gregory was not able to reflect on what they had found and why the surgery was necessary (that is never a good sign). What got my attention about him was the fact that a steroid injection in his foot resolved his symptoms for some time.

After examining him I decided to get an x-ray of his jaw. My thought was something that may be in his neck could possibly be responsible for his symptoms in the right jaw/neck area. The x-ray confirmed what I was thinking all along. His stylohyoid ligament that typically should not be visible on an x-ray was visible (they looked like two chopsticks going down into his throat).

Calcification of the ligament (as seen in the x-ray below), along with the symptoms he presented, warranted a diagnosis of Eagles syndrome, which is a rare condition characterized by sudden, sharp, nerve-like pain in the jawbone and joint, back of the throat, and base of the tongue. Treatment would be injection of steroid into the area or removal of the ligament.

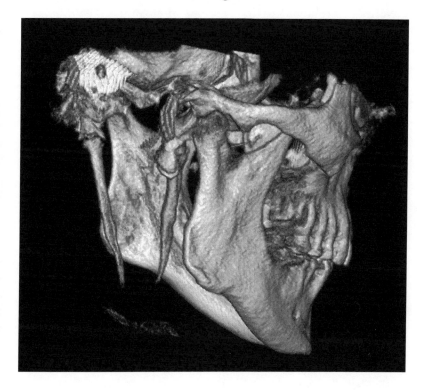

My working diagnosis was myalgia on both sides, which was probably due to his chronic history of teeth grinding, capsulitis of both temporomandibular joints, and he was already diagnosed with obstructive sleep apnea (adult).

Due to the nature of feeling that there was a foreign body in the throat and constant need to clear his throat, and radiographic presence of bilateral calcification of his stylohyoid ligament, Gregory presents with signs and symptoms of Eagles syndrome.

When we gave him the diagnosis he started to cry, followed by his wife. I really felt a bit uncomfortable and baffled. I wondered, did I say something wrong? What is going? Once they got themselves together Gregory said, "finally an answer" to what he was experiencing.

They were both relieved. After 30 years of chasing his symptoms, and fears of the worst possible outcome of cancer, they had something to work off of. From here we referred him to an ENT to have a discussion on his surgical options.

As you can see from the outcomes for these patients, diagnosis and treatment was vital in ensuring they were able to live their day-to-day lives without pain and other complications. Pain and TMD take a toll on your life, and can disrupt your daily routines, so don't wait idly by as the pain worsens--contact a dentist who specializes in craniofacial pain and TMD today.

Alternative TMD Relief

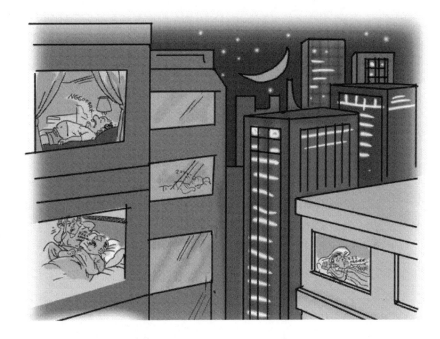

Treatment doesn't always mean medications or appliances--there is a variety of alternatives available for relief. If you would rather skip medication or the purchase of a device, there might be some alternative treatment options available, including essential oils, stress relief options and physical therapy.

However, it is important to remember that alternative options might not work for certain cases of craniofacial pain, jaw pain and TMD. Please talk to your dentist or physician for further guidance.

Here is how these options might help in providing you with proper relief from jaw pain and discomfort.

1. **Essential Oils** - particularly useful in the management of chronic pain, such as arthritis or headaches. What makes essential oils even more special is that they help to remedy at least some of the conditions that caused the pain. For example, peppermint essential oil is used on aching muscles and headaches. Peppermint not only improves blood circulation to the area, but also helps to reduce the inflammation that causes the pain.

2. **Stress Relief Options** - relaxation techniques can help to calm your mind, reduce stress hormones in your blood, relax your muscles, and elevate your sense of well-being. By actively using stress relief and relaxation exercises, you can experience long-term changes in your body to counteract the harmful effects of stress, such as chronic pain.

3. **Physical Therapy** - managing chronic pain by administering physical therapy options play an important role in relief. Physical therapy might include strengthening and flexibility exercises, manual therapy, posture awareness, and body mechanics instructions. This is another natural option for finding relief from pain.

Throughout this book we have looked at the definition of craniofacial pain and temporomandibular joint disorder (TMD). We've also discussed how some pain experienced can be felt in the ears or face when it is really caused by the TMJ. Understanding referred pain can help in improving diagnosis and treatment planning.

While there are various treatments available, it is important to find the best one for your individual case. Some patients might experience relief through at-home remedies, but many still require treatment provided from a dentist for physician.

And most importantly, if you take anything from reading this book, remember to educate yourself! I cannot put enough emphasis on this. The more you know, the better you can protect yourself from further pain and harm.

Meet the Authors

This book was a collaborative effort from Dr. Mayoor Patel and Sara Berg. While not super heroes, this dynamic Dentist – Writer duo has been able to bring to light important information in the area of Craniofacial Pain and TMD. Why? Because a dentist has all of the knowledge, but may not always know how to put it down on paper in words that are easily understood by most patients.

In this team effort, Dr. Patel and Sara discuss the importance of diagnosis and treatment so you can finally say "goodbye" to pain and "hello" to daily enjoyment of your life. Educational books don't have to be boring, which is why this Dentist and Writer teamed up in creating "Take a Bite Out of TMD." We hope you enjoyed the book!

Dr. Mayoor Patel, DDS, MS

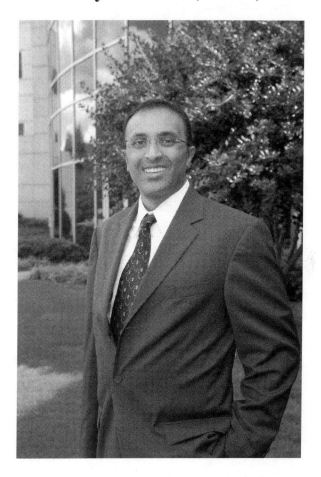

After receiving his dental degree from the University of Tennessee in 1994, Dr. Mayoor Patel went on to complete a one-year residency in Advanced Education in General Dentistry (AEGD). Dr. Mayoor Patel is a Diplomate in the American Board of Orofacial Pain, Craniofacial Pain, Dental Sleep Medicine and Craniofacial Dental Sleep Medicine.

Dr. Patel has also earned a Fellowship in the American Academy of Orofacial Pain, Craniofacial Pain, the International College of Craniomandibular Orthopedics and the Academy of General Dentistry. Additionally, Dr. Patel is the second dentist in the

United States that has fulfilled the necessary requirements and is a registered polysomnographic technologist.

Dr. Patel currently serves with Tufts University, Augusta University and the Atlanta Sleep School. His practice is located in Atlanta, GA and is limited to Facial Pain, TMJ Disorders and Sleep disordered breathing.

To learn more about Dr. Patel, please visit www.mpateldds.com.

Sara Berg

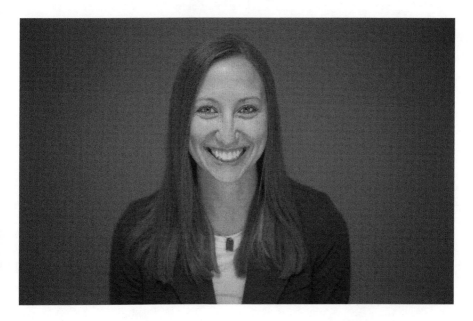

A versatile writer who has been known to wear multiple hats on numerous occasions, Sara Berg received her Bachelor's Degree in English from Bradley University in Peoria, IL.

After graduation, Sara took her degree and ran with her love of writing. She has worked as a Copywriter and Content Manager at Officite, LLC, a web development firm for the healthcare industry.

Four years later, Sara transitioned into her role as a Content Marketing Associate for Empire Today, LLC—yes, the carpet company. Go ahead and sing the jingle (we know you want to). She then went on to become a Content Marketing Manager before transitioning into a full-time freelance Writer, Editor and Content Specialist.

Because she wanted to get as much experience as possible in different industries, Sara began her freelance writing career with an open field for writing. From her experience writing for all medical areas at Officite,

Sara began honing in her expertise and creativity in the area of Sleep Dentistry and Craniofacial Pain, and continues her freelance writing for a variety of clients within the dental industry.

To learn more about Sara Berg and her experience, please visit www.saraiceberg.com.

Made in United States
Orlando, FL
15 December 2023